A Year's Worth of Yellow

By Emma Rose Sparrow

Publish Date: February 13, 2015

Editor-in-Chief: Connor Chagnon
Sterling Elle Publishing
Bradford, Massachusetts
ISBN-10: 1517401399
ISBN-13: 978-1517401399

A YEAR'S WORTH OF YELLOW

An Emma Rose Sparrow Book

A YEAR'S WORTH OF YELLOW is a collection of amazing photos - with accompanying text - that have one thing in common: the color yellow!

You may be surprised to find out how many different ways yellow shows up in the world. From yellow sea creatures that cling to coral to rustic yellow painted homes in Greece, this book brings the color yellow to life.

If you are an adult bookworm who enjoys exquisite photos, this book is for you!

It is hoped that you find this book worthy of adding to your collection.

Enjoy your read!

EMMA ROSE SPARROW

OTHER BOOKS IN THIS SERIES
BY EMMA ROSE SPARROW

A Potpourri of Pink

A Bevy of Blue

A Gathering of Green

A Parcel of Purple

A Reservoir of Red

A World of White

An Ocean of Orange

EMMA ROSE SPARROW

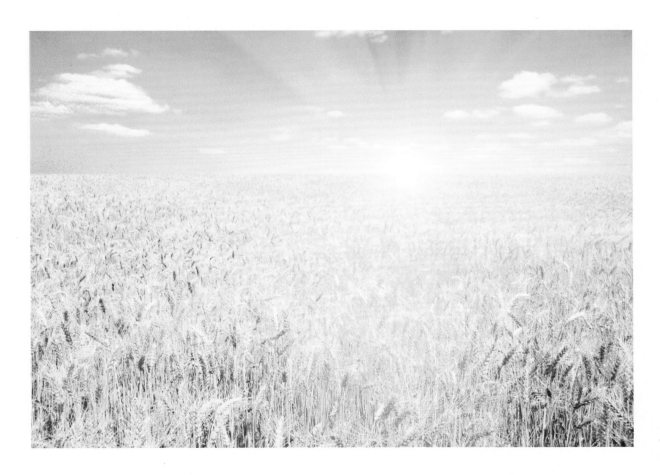

A golden yellow sunset over a gorgeous wheat field.

EMMA ROSE SPARROW

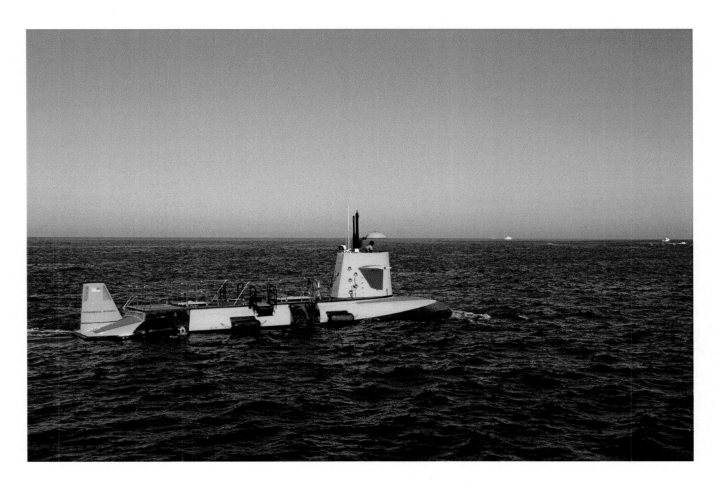

This yellow submarine has a glass bottom that allows tourists to view the marine life off the coast of California.

EMMA ROSE SPARROW

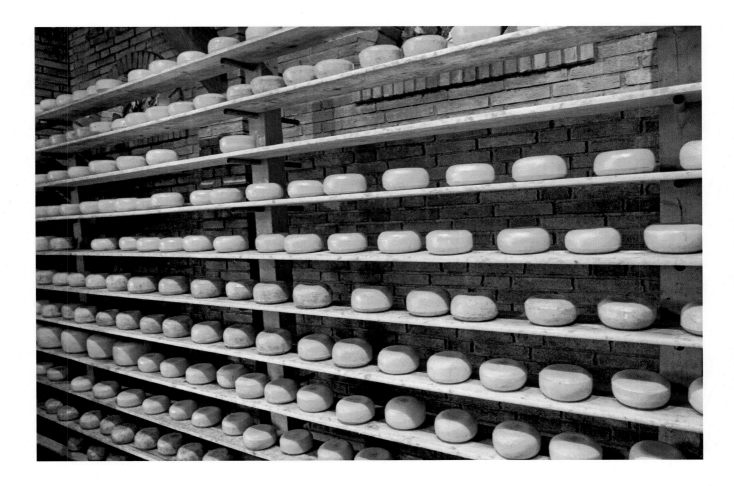

These endless rows of yellow cheese can be found at a cheese factory in Holland.

EMMA ROSE SPARROW

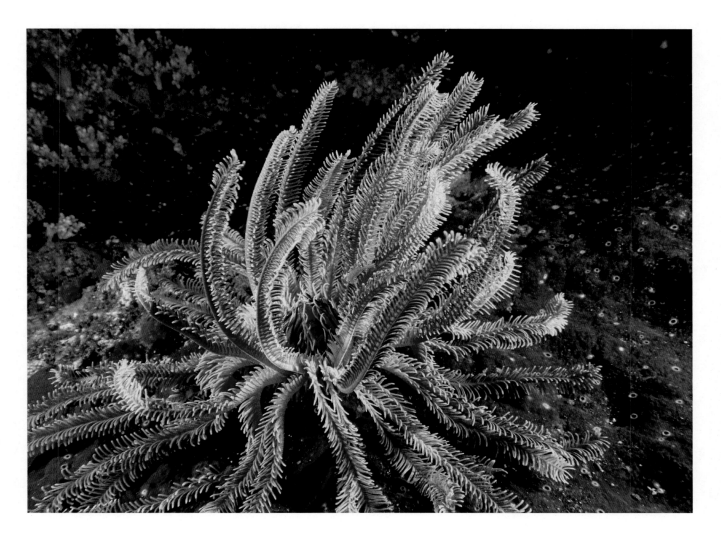

This beautiful yellow coral thrives off the coast of Indonesia.

EMMA ROSE SPARROW

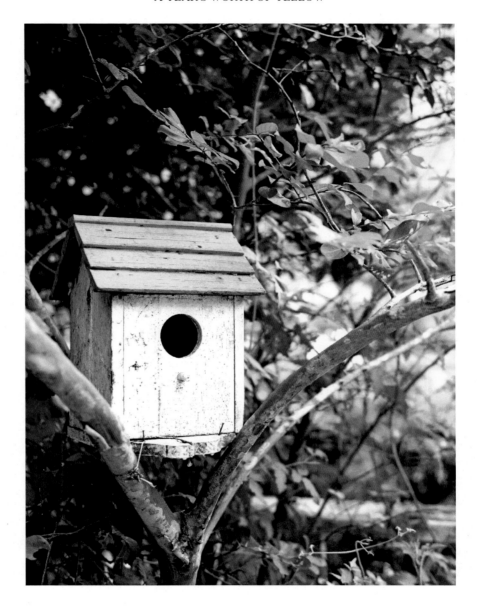

This homemade wooden birdhouse with its pale yellow roof
is nested on a young sapling.

EMMA ROSE SPARROW

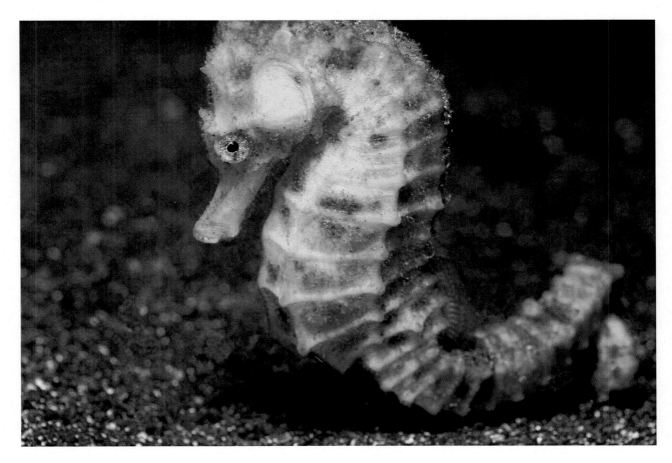

This cute little sea creature is a Yellow Common Seahorse.

EMMA ROSE SPARROW

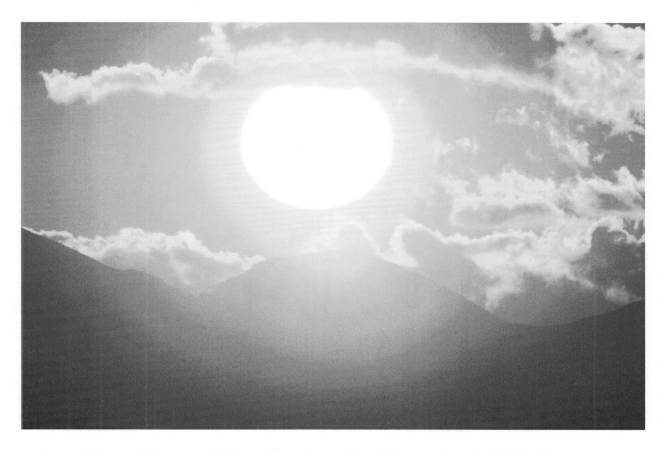

The yellow sunlight reflecting off of these clouds is glorious.

EMMA ROSE SPARROW

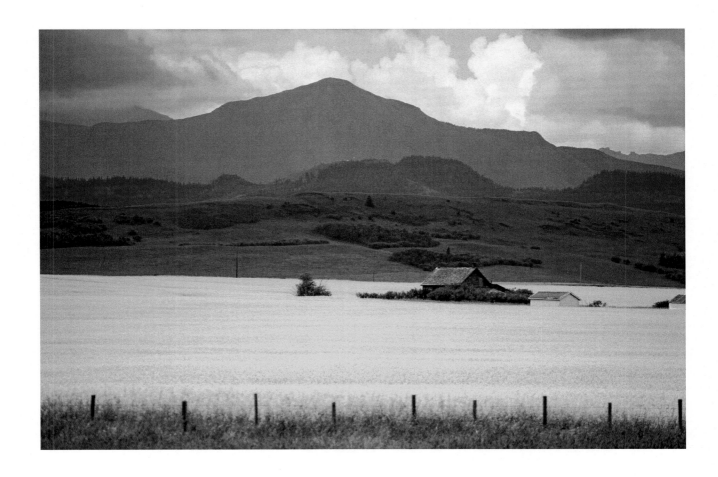

A farm house surrounded by fields of yellow canola plants.

EMMA ROSE SPARROW

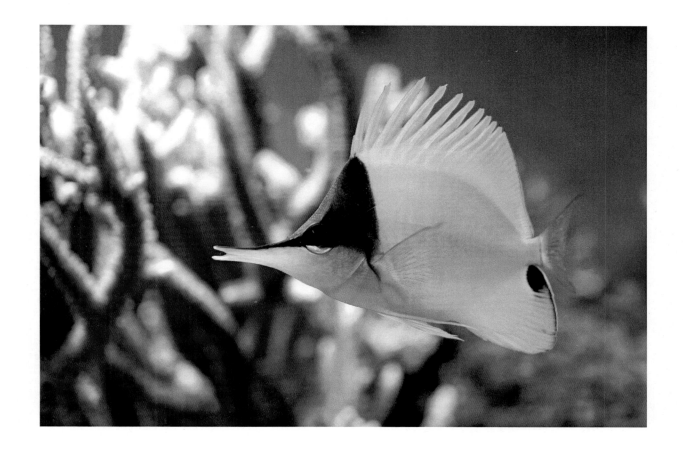

This amusing fish is called the Yellow Longnose Butterflyfish.

EMMA ROSE SPARROW

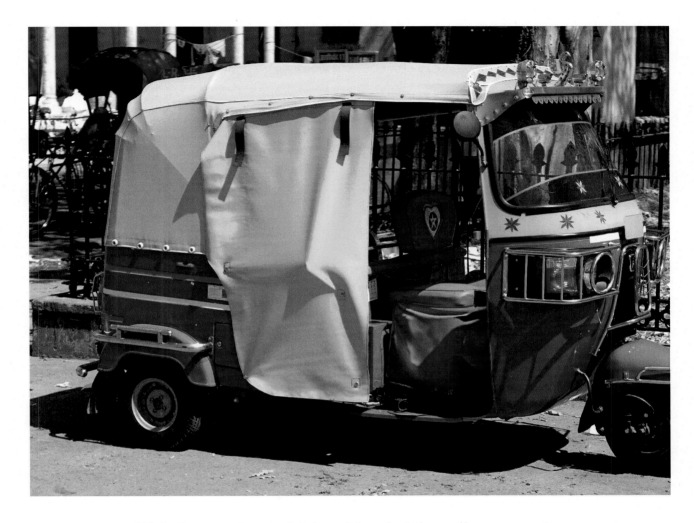

This interesting vehicle with a bright yellow covering
is a 'rickshaw' taxi in India .

EMMA ROSE SPARROW

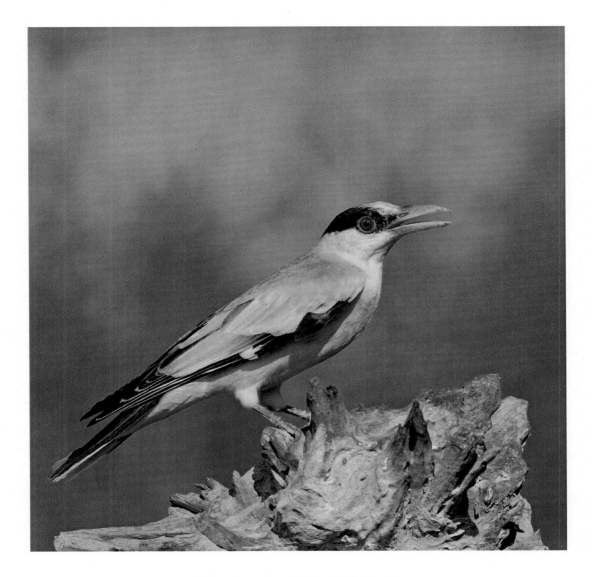

Black-naped Oriole bird.
Despite the name, this bird's nape (neck) is bright yellow.

EMMA ROSE SPARROW

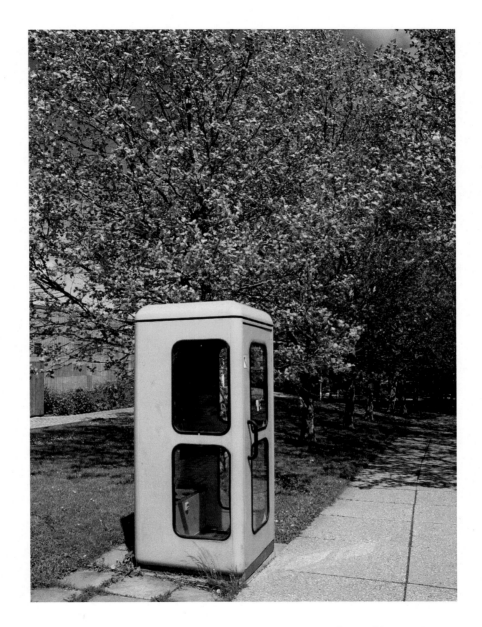

This yellow telephone booth sits near a sidewalk in Germany.

EMMA ROSE SPARROW

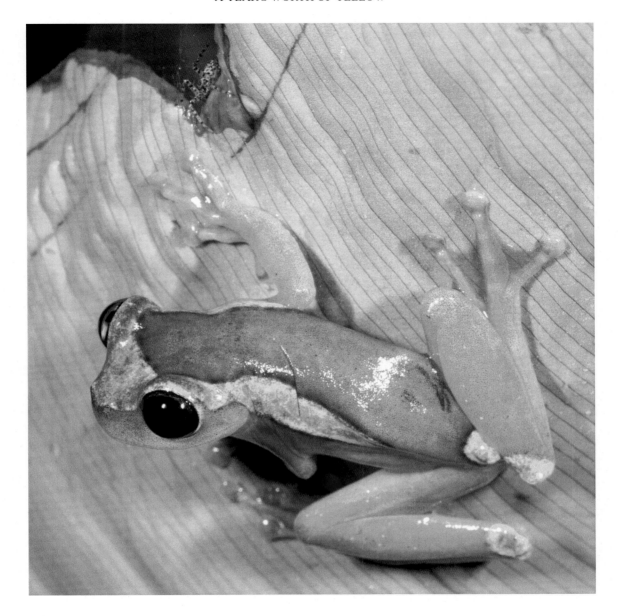

This is the Upper Amazon Tree Frog.
It is a bright yellow frog that lives in tropical jungles.

EMMA ROSE SPARROW

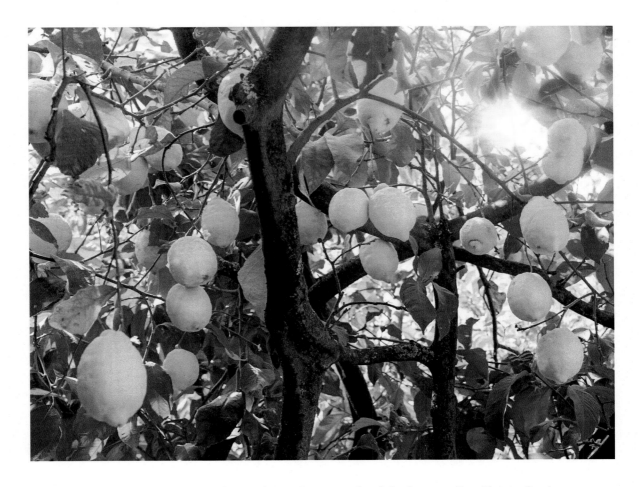

This lemon tree found in Greece holds lots of yellow fruit.
In Greece, lemons are the 2nd most widely produced fruit (oranges are #1).

EMMA ROSE SPARROW

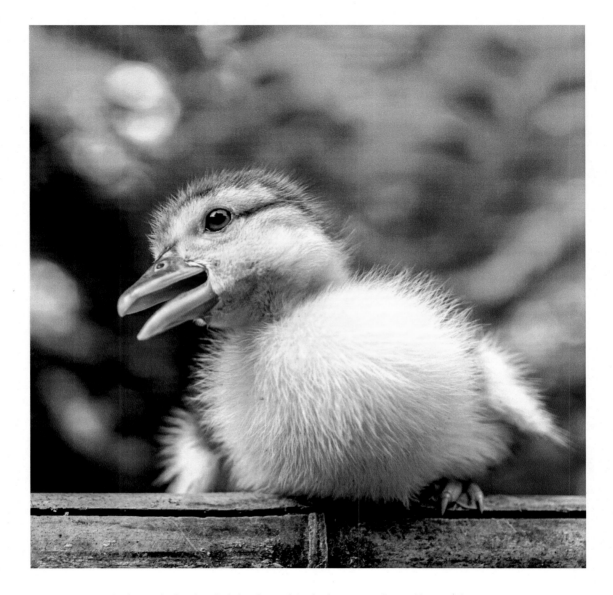

This delightful baby duck has soft yellow down.
This will be replaced with white feathers as he matures.

EMMA ROSE SPARROW

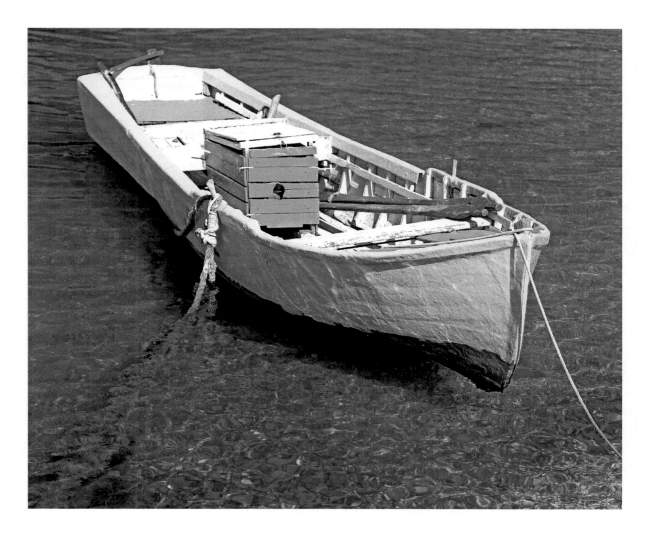

A hand painted yellow boat is docked at a lake in Bulgaria.

EMMA ROSE SPARROW

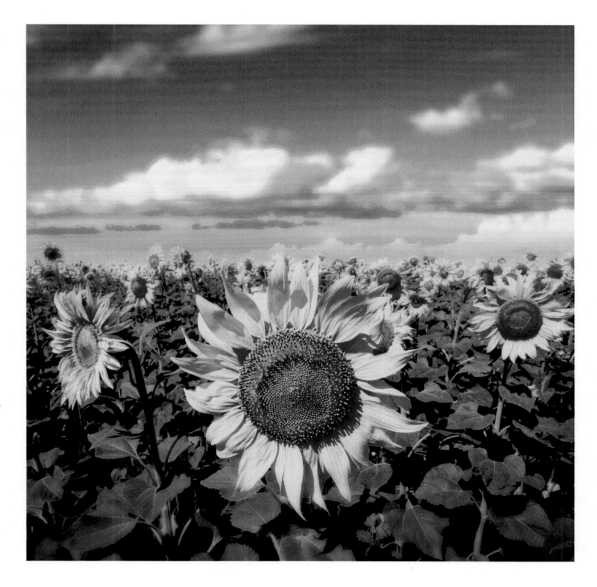

These splendid bright yellow sunflowers make for a stunning photo.
Sunflowers can grow up to 10 feet high.

EMMA ROSE SPARROW

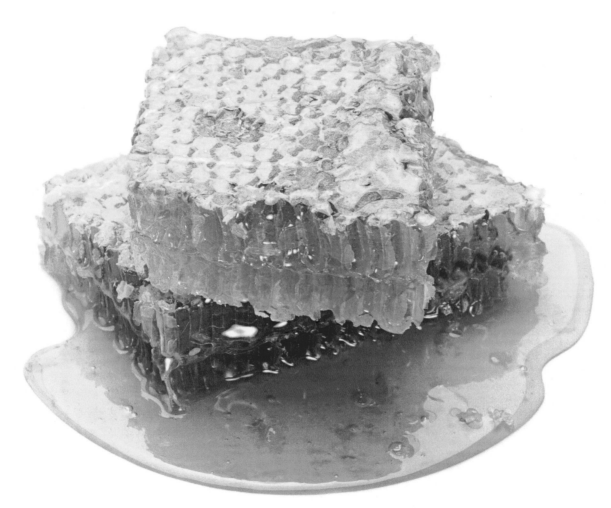

These syrupy honeycombs look tempting with
sweet yellow honey packed into them.

EMMA ROSE SPARROW

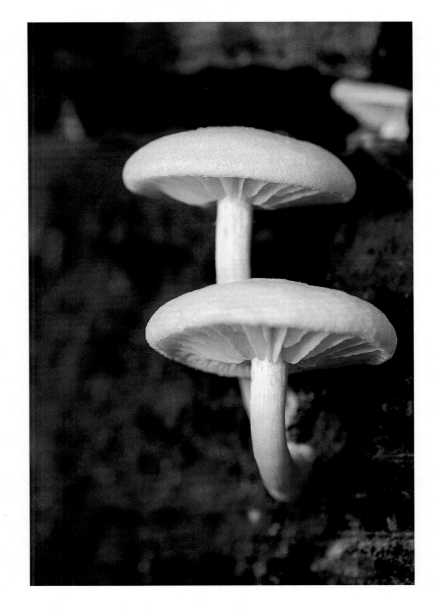

These are Butter Waxcap mushrooms.
While these are edible, they are too fragile to be used for cooking.

EMMA ROSE SPARROW

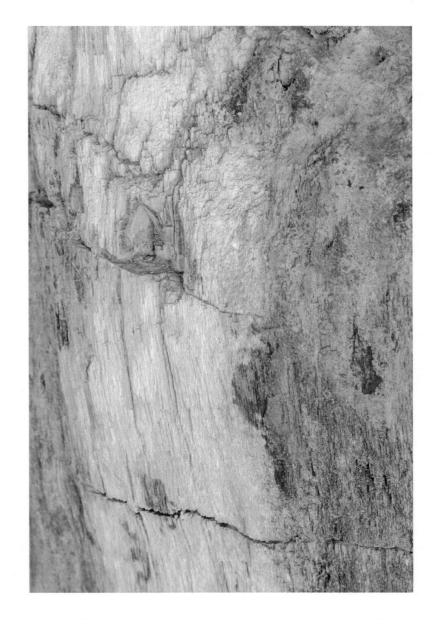

This yellow rock wall, with dashes of bright red, can be found in Thailand.

EMMA ROSE SPARROW

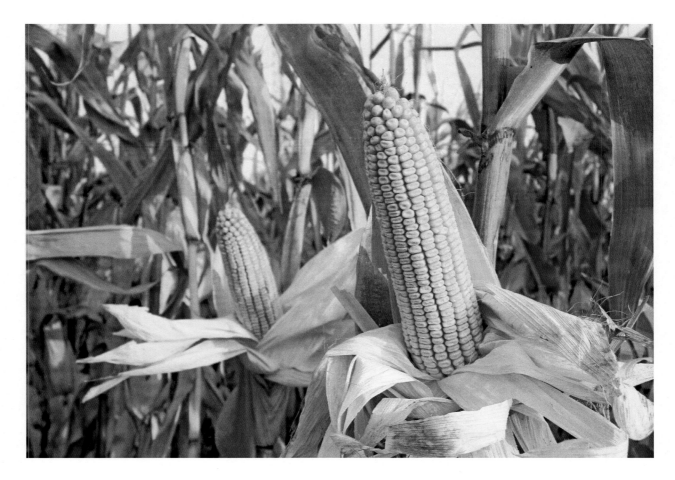

Corn is native to the Americas.
This yellow vegetable was first introduced to Europe in the late 15th century.

EMMA ROSE SPARROW

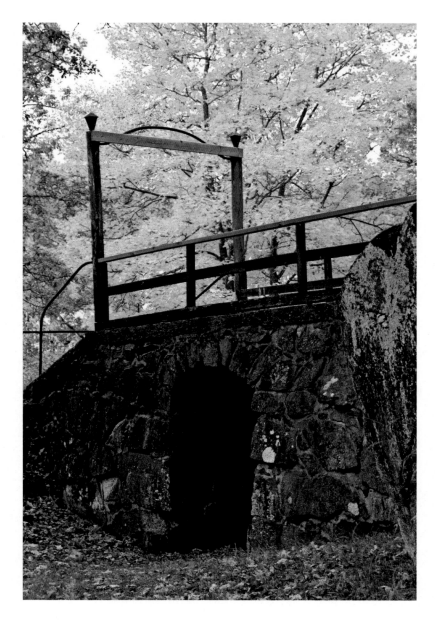

This rock overpass has a background of gorgeous yellow foliage.

EMMA ROSE SPARROW

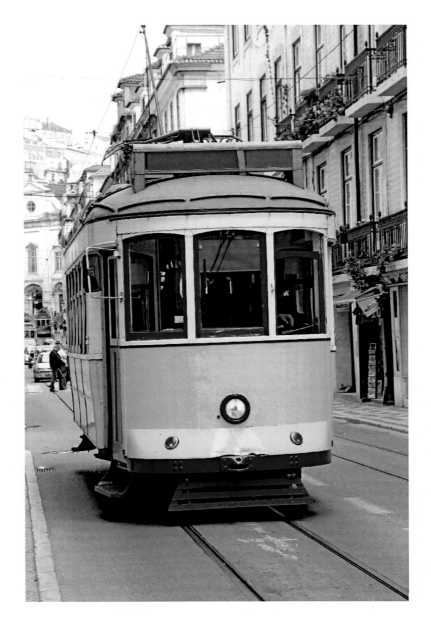

This yellow trolley car is used to transport riders in Portugal.

EMMA ROSE SPARROW

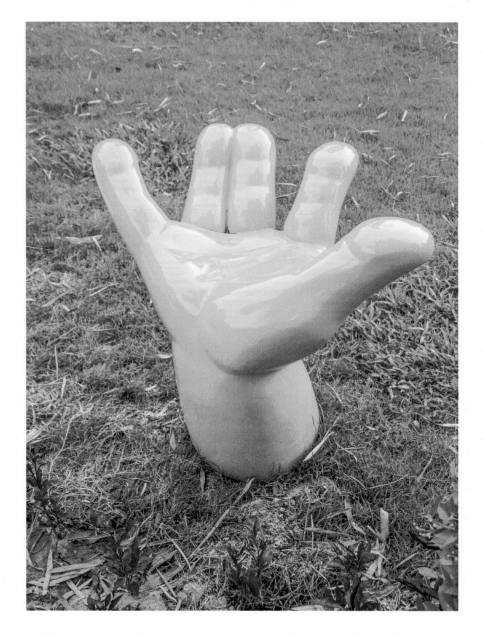

This large yellow hand is actually a garden chair!

EMMA ROSE SPARROW

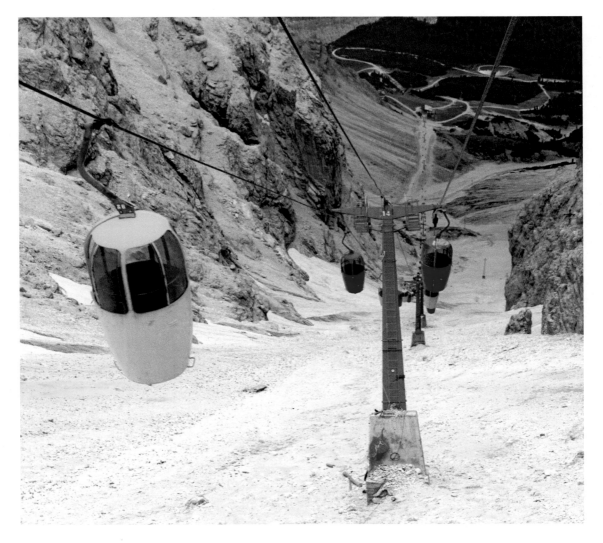

This cheerful yellow cable car is just one of the many brightly colored pods that bring people up a mountain in Italy.

EMMA ROSE SPARROW

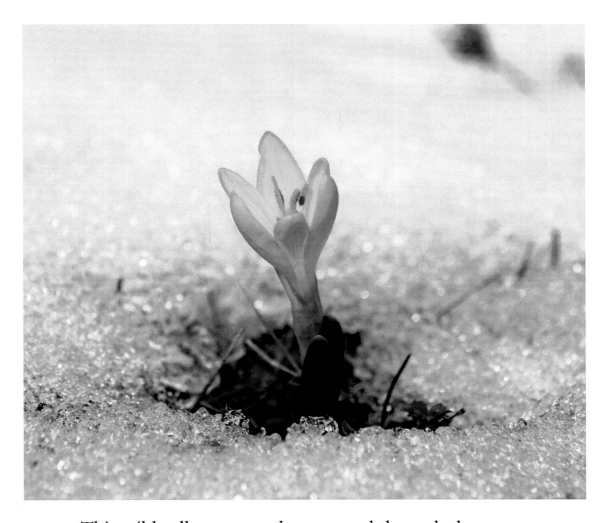

This wild yellow crocus has popped through the snow.
These spring flowers tend to come up early,
announcing that winter is almost done.

EMMA ROSE SPARROW

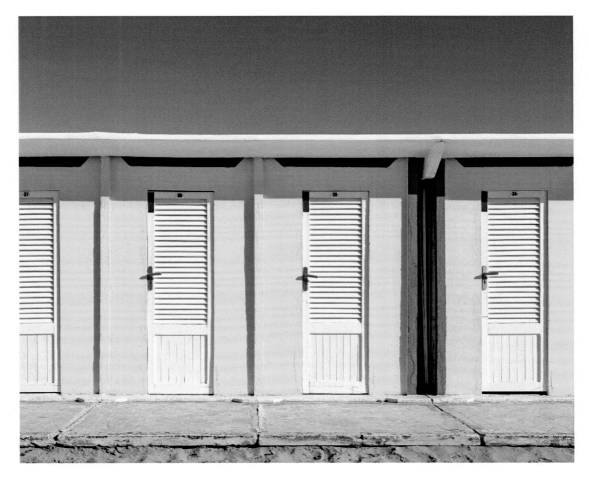

You can find these bright yellow beach huts in Rimini, a coastal city in Italy.

EMMA ROSE SPARROW

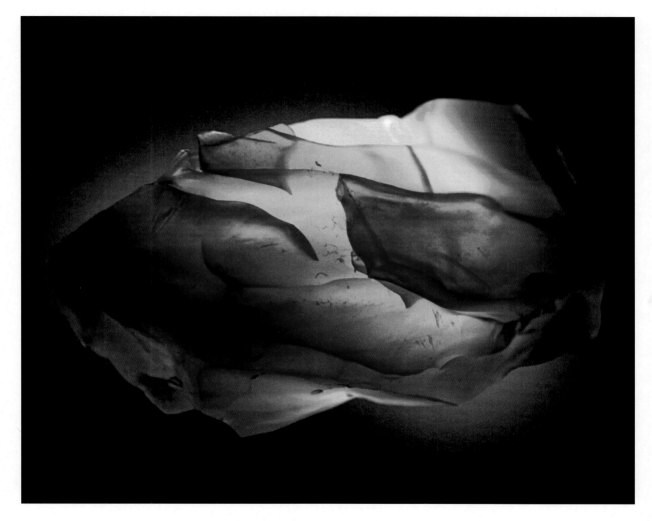

Opal can be found in many colors.
Yellow opal, pictured here, is also referred to as the 'Stone of Comfort'.

EMMA ROSE SPARROW

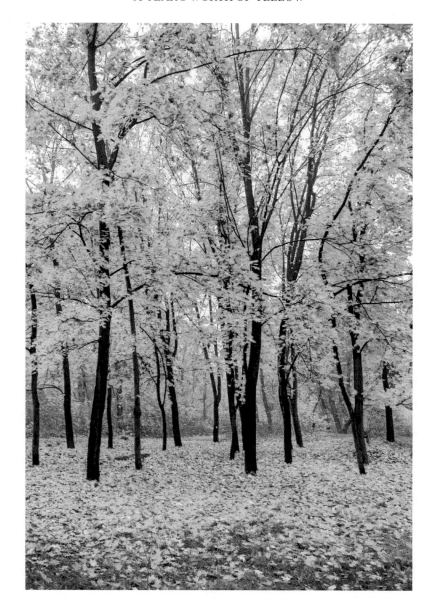

These dazzling yellow leaves show how lovely autumn can be.

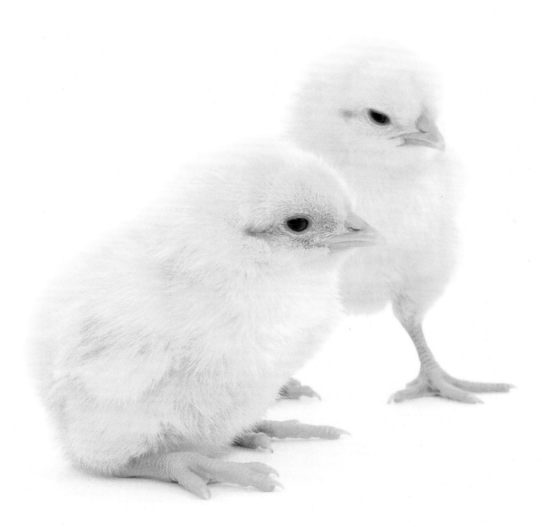

These pale yellow baby chicks are only 4 days old.

EMMA ROSE SPARROW

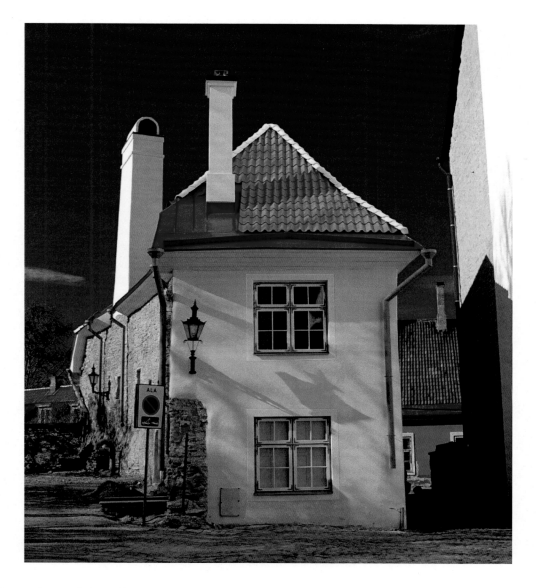

This cheerful yellow house can be found in a historic part of Tallinn,
a city in Estonia.

EMMA ROSE SPARROW

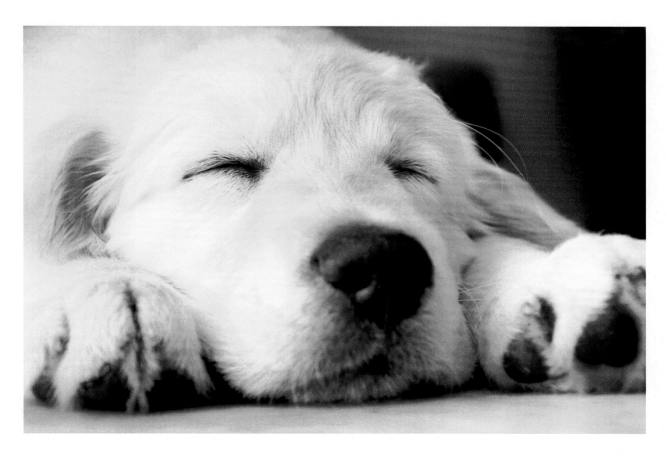

A Golden Retriever fast asleep.
These pale yellow dogs are known for being intelligent, friendly and easy to train.

EMMA ROSE SPARROW

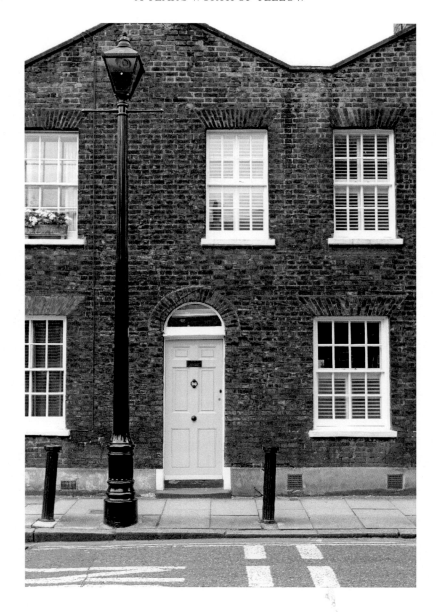

This bright yellow door stands out against a brick house in London.

EMMA ROSE SPARROW

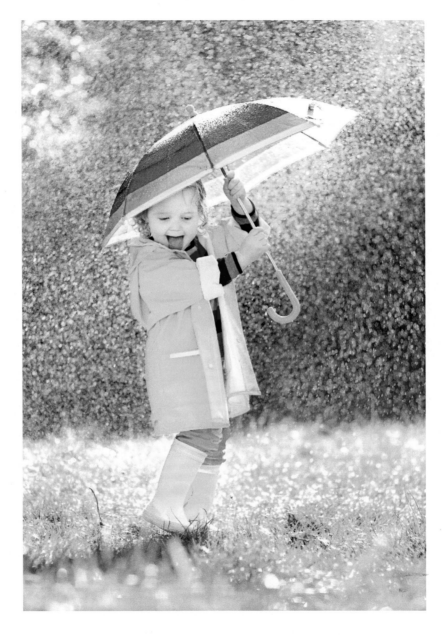

A young girl enjoys a sun shower in her matching yellow raincoat and boots.

EMMA ROSE SPARROW

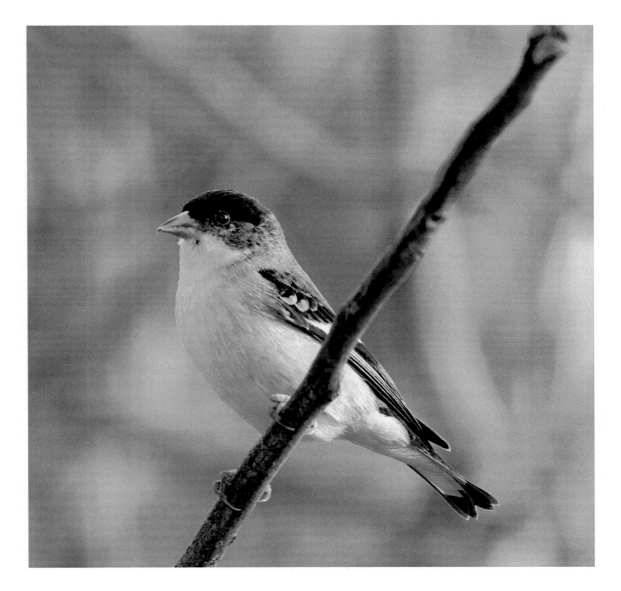

This yellow bird is the Lesser Goldfinch songbird.
When it sings, it changes pitch from high (teeeyeee) to low (teeeyooo).

EMMA ROSE SPARROW

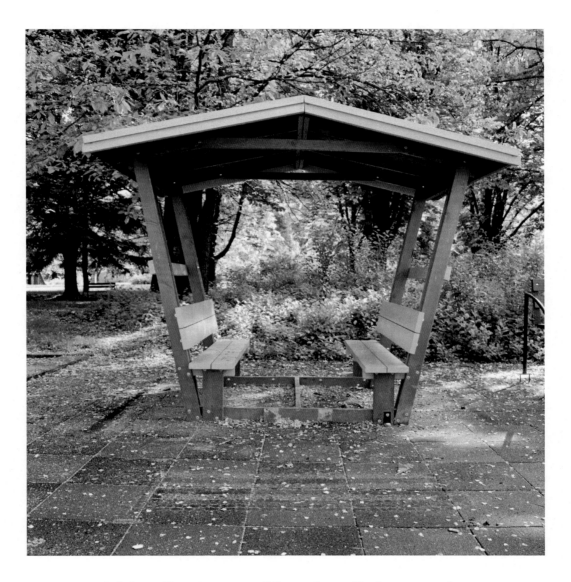

This yellow covered bench, called a pergola,
provides a shaded resting area in a Georgia park.

EMMA ROSE SPARROW

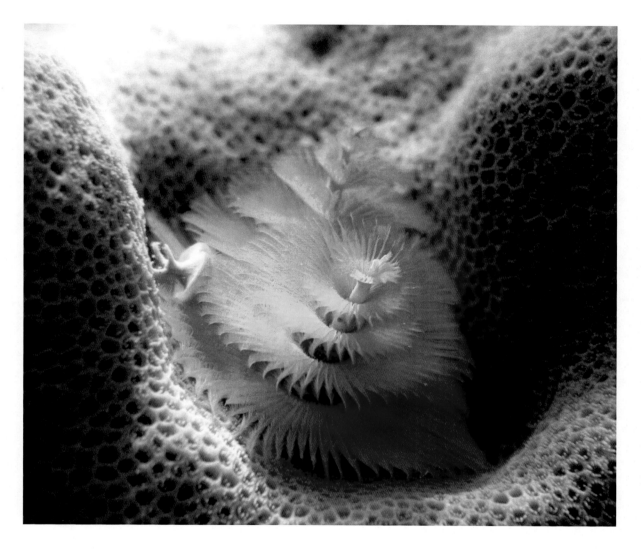

The yellow Christmas tree worm, an unusual sea creature, lives on coral reefs.

EMMA ROSE SPARROW

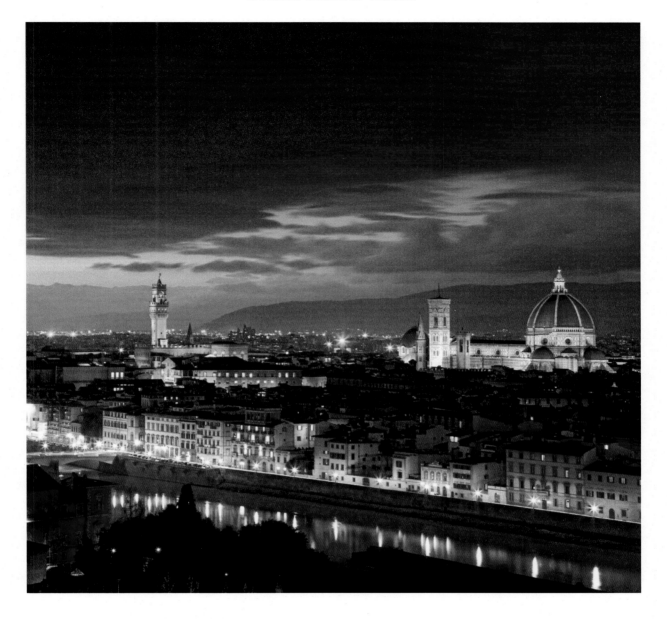

At night, yellow lights shine throughout Florence, Italy.

EMMA ROSE SPARROW

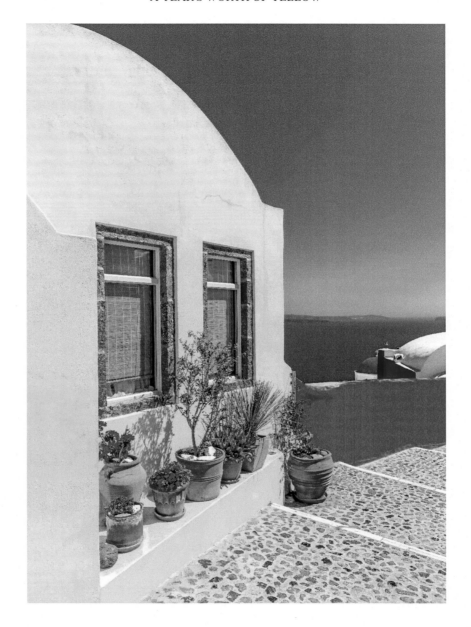

On Santorini island, Greece, it is common for homes to be brightly painted.
This lively yellow house is a perfect example.

EMMA ROSE SPARROW

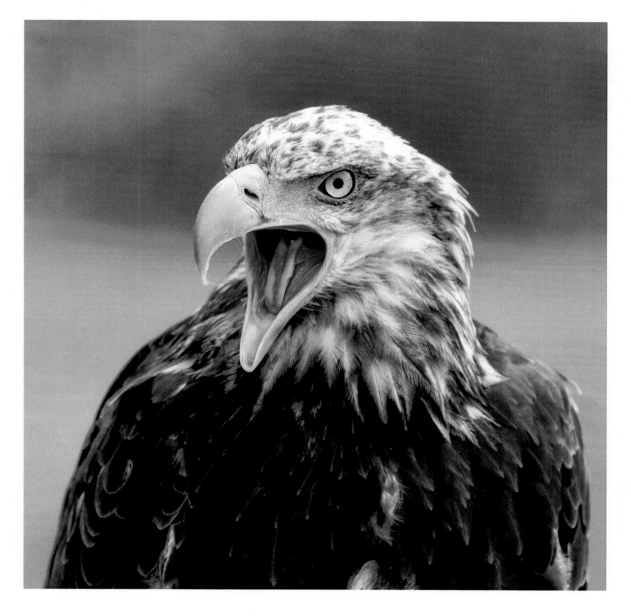

The American Bald Eagle builds the largest nest of any North American bird.
Both its beak and irises are yellow.

EMMA ROSE SPARROW

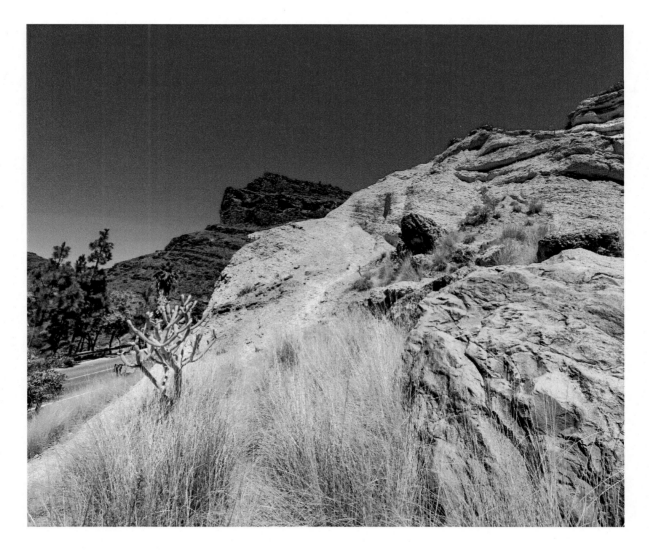

This wild yellow landscape can be found in the Canary Islands.

EMMA ROSE SPARROW

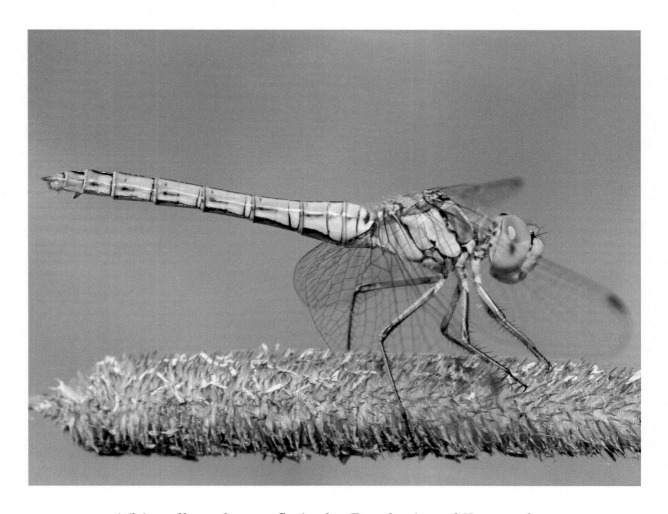

This yellow dragonfly is the Band-winged Dragonlet.
In China, the dragonfly symbolizes harmony and good luck.
In Japan, it symbolizes both summer and autumn.

EMMA ROSE SPARROW

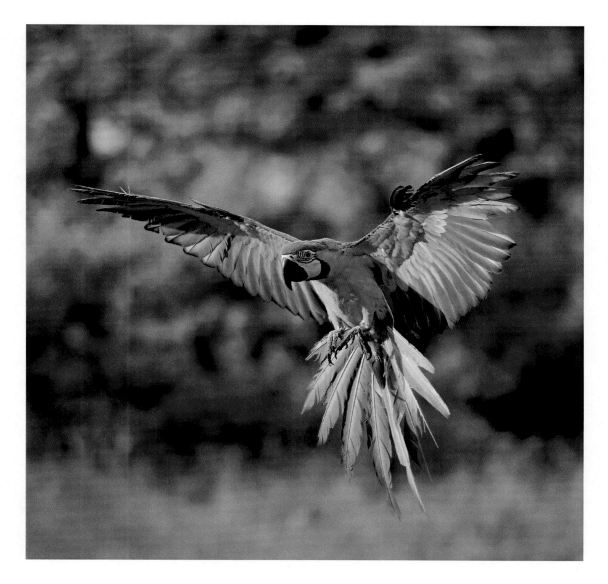

This blue-and-yellow Macaw prepares to land.

EMMA ROSE SPARROW

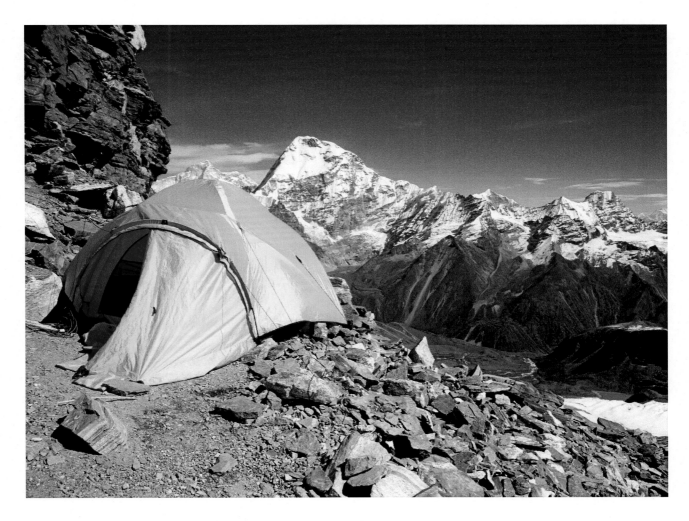

This bright yellow tent marks the camping site of climbers on Mt. Everest.

EMMA ROSE SPARROW

OTHER BOOKS IN THIS SERIES
BY EMMA ROSE SPARROW

A Potpourri of Pink

A Bevy of Blue

A Gathering of Green

A Parcel of Purple

A Reservoir of Red

A World of White

An Ocean of Orange

Photo Credits

The artist/source credits for the photos in this book are listed in the order in which they appear:

Skylines/Shutterstock.com
Rodolfo Arpia/ Shutterstock.com
BESTWEB/Shutterstock.com
Teerinvata/Shutterstock.com
Johnson76/Shutterstock.com
Andaman/Shutterstock.com
UMB-O/Shutterstock.com
Robert Crum/Shutterstock.com
Dobermaraner/Shutterstock.com
nevenm/Shutterstock.com
BOONCHUAY
PROMJIAM/Shutterstock.com
Flori0/Shutterstock.com
Dr. Morley Read/Shutterstock.com
haraldmuc/Shutterstock.com
24Novembers/Shutterstock.com
Jaroslav Moravcik/Shutterstock.com
Ase/Shutterstock.com
Valentyn Volkov/Shutterstock.com
joharhu/Shutterstock.com
KobchaiMa/Shutterstock.com
branislavpudar/Shutterstock.com
Linda Z/Shutterstock.com

karnizz/Shutterstock.com
Nuk2013/Shutterstock.com
Florin Stana/Shutterstock.com
Lusine/Shutterstock.com
Ppictures/Shutterstock.com
Albert Russ/Shutterstock.com
Pavel Vakhrushev/Shutterstock.com
Tsekhmister/Shutterstock.com
Raimundo79/Shutterstock.com
Milosz Aniol/Shutterstock.com
Cantemir Olaru/Shutterstock.com
FamVeld/Shutterstock.com
Birdiegal/Shutterstock.com
eenevski/Shutterstock.com
LauraD/Shutterstock.com
SJ Travel Photo and
Vid/Shutterstock..com
imagIN.gr photography/Shutterstock.com
Pal Teravagimov/Shutterstock.com
Mr. Green/Shutterstock.com
Lydeke Bosch/Shutterstock.com
Stanislav Duben/Shutterstock.com
Yongyut Kumsri/Shutterstock.com